Diabetes Guide:

Simply Tips For Simly Life With Diabetes

Table of Content

Introduction

The general public has been surrounded by medications and frightening tools used to treat diabetes; therefore, it's no wonder most people are terrified when they're diagnosed with it. However, a diagnosis of diabetes, no matter what type, is not a death sentence. It's merely a malfunctioning of the pancreas that must be corrected with either diet, medication or both. A lifestyle change is in order, but people diagnosed with this disease can live long, healthy lives.

The first step to diagnosing diabetes is seeing a doctor for a glucose intolerance test. This test may require fasting, but not always. It depends on which type of diabetes the doctors are looking for. The good news is for people over the age of twenty, the doctors are most likely looking for type 2 diabetes, which is the less severe of the two. Do not panic if a diagnosis of type 1 diabetes comes back, though because it is just as manageable as type 2.

The second step, after the diagnosis, is assessing the patient's meal plan and their daily lifestyle. People diagnosed with this illness are usually overweight due to unhealthy eating habits and lack of exercise. Sometimes, just changing those two factors can reverse some of the damages done by the disease already.

The third step is making sure the patient is educated enough about the disease and understands their medication and their new plan. This is the phase where doctors make sure the patient is not falling into depression or needs help learning new coping skills.

The final step is living with the disease. This book will briefly describe the different types of diabetes and the tests run to diagnose them. Then it will go on to describe how a patient's new lifestyle will look. Finally, it will briefly go over how to cope with the stress of managing diabetes.

Management of diabetes may seem impossible at first with all the information the doctor might be providing. Keeping track medications and supplements can lead to an ever riskier problem that forgetting to exercise once; stress. Chronic stress can cause severe problems in people with diabetes and should be avoided at all costs. It can lead to much more serious health problems, but this book will teach people with diabetes how to manage their daily lives and give them some helpful information on choosing medications with the help of a doctor.

The first thing people think they need to do is cut all carbs and sugars from their diet. This is untrue and unsafe! The chapter on diet management will discuss healthy portions and choices when a person is trying to change their diet to fit their lifestyle. Thinking about diabetes as just a lifestyle change is much easier and positive than thinking about it as a debilitating illness.

The chapter on herbal management will discuss several different herbal remedies that are used to treat diabetes. These are the herbs that have been proven with scientific studies to help; although, there are a lot of herbal remedies out there that claim to help but have not been proven. It is important to discuss herbal remedy interactions with prescription medications with a doctor to be absolutely sure, as hypoglycemia is a common side-effect that can be dangerous.

When the body is stress chronically, it will start to break down. Let's face it, being diagnosed with a disease that will permanently affect one's life is stressful, but it doesn't have to be forever. Learning how to manage the disease and manage stress will help you live a happier, more fulfilling life. Anyone can benefit from less stress in their life, and there are numerous ways to dispel of it.

A routine is basically the end result of learning how to manage all these different aspects of your life with diabetes. It's not going to come easy at first, but planning everything out step by step and having a comprehensive guide to the different things that need to be addressed is a great start. Remember, a routine is made of habits, and it takes time to build these.

Learning how to manage diabetes will not happen overnight, but having the information at your fingertips will make it that much easier.

Chapter 1 – Understanding Diabetes

When faced with a diagnosis of diabetes, the majority of people understand it means they have a surplus of glucose in their bloodstream. This surplus of glucose occurs when the pancreas no longer functions properly. While this is true, diabetes can be caused by a multitude of problems. Depending upon the type, eating healthy and monitoring blood glucose levels may not be enough. It is imperative the patient understands what type of diabetes they have and how they can control it. More importantly, knowing how the pancreas functions to better understand why diabetes is occurring explains how to control it.

The pancreas is what controls the levels of insulin, a hormone in the body. When a person consumes sugar, their pancreas turns this sugar into insulin, which then moves nutrients such as sugar into cells of the body's tissue. These cells use glucose and other nutrients as a source of energy to function properly. Without these nutrients, they cannot renew themselves or protect the body from infection.

Classic symptoms of diabetes can be related to so many other illnesses, the only way to properly diagnose it is a blood test. A doctor may conduct more than one blood test over a certain amount of time to be sure the patient is suffering from low blood glucose and to determine the type. Some symptoms patients may exhibit are increased thirst, frequent urination, extreme hunger, unexplained weight loss, ketones in the urine, fatigue, irritability, blurred vision, slow-healing sores, and frequent infections. All of these symptoms occur because the insulin is no longer carrying sugar and other nutrients to the cells.

When diagnosing diabetes, the first thing a doctor will do is examine the symptoms. If they suspect low or high blood sugar is occurring, they will begin to run tests. The first test run will be a fasting plasma glucose test. It is an easy test to run and relatively inexpensive compared to other tests. The FPG test requires the patient to fast for at least eight hours before the blood is drawn. Once the test results are back, usually within a day or two depending upon the lab it was sent to, the doctor will inform the patient of the results.

For the FPG test, a fasting blood glucose should be between seventy to one hundred milligrams per deciliter for normal people. If it is abnormal, one hundred and twenty-six milligrams per deciliter or above, then the doctor will order another test to be sure. If the patient has a normal FPG test, but they are still exhibiting signs of diabetes, the doctor may order a casual plasma glucose test for diabetes.

The casual plasma glucose test or CPG measures the amount of glucose in a person's blood regardless of when they last ate. Meaning, the patient does not abstain from eating before the blood is drawn. A result of two hundred milligrams per deciliter or greater will hint at diabetes. The doctor will perform another test at a later date to confirm.

The reason a doctor may perform the CPG test is because the patient may not develop high blood glucose levels until they have eaten. Some people may seem normal until they eat a meal, and then their glucose levels will spike dramatically. That is why they may come back with a normal FPG test, but an abnormal CPG test.

Once faced with a diagnosis of diabetes, patients may go through three more tests throughout their lifetime to monitor potential health risks. These tests include the A1C test, blood pressure monitoring, and cholesterol levels monitoring. These tests determine if an individual is responding well to their medication and changes in their diet they have made.

The A1C test measures the average blood sugar level over the past three months. It is different from the blood sugar level checks a person does each day because it tells the doctor whether or not the condition is worsening. If the blood sugar rises over time, the heart, blood vessels, kidneys, feet and eyes can be affected dramatically. The normal range for someone with diabetes is a rating below seven. However, the doctor will better be able to tell someone what their level should be.

Blood pressure can be monitored by a doctor or an individual can buy a blood pressure monitoring kit at a local drug store. Blood pressure is the force of blood against the wall of the blood vessels. It is imperative to keep blood pressure below 140/90 for people with diabetes. If this number is too high, it makes the heart work too hard and can cause a heart attack, stroke, or damage to the kidneys and eyes.

Even people without diabetes should monitor their cholesterol as this is an important part of modern day health. There are two different kinds of cholesterol in the body: LDL and HDL. Bad cholesterol is LDL, which can build up and clog blood vessels. This may cause a heart attack or stroke. Good cholesterol, HDL, removes bad cholesterol from the blood vessels. Anyone over the age of forty should have their cholesterol levels checked, but people with diabetes are prone to having out of whack levels.

If diabetes is not monitored, there are numerous health problems that will occur. People who do not take their medication or change their diet may experience heart attacks, strokes, eye problems that may lead to trouble seeing or going blind, pain, tingling, numbness in the hands and feet that is caused by nerve damage, kidney problems that may result in failure, and teeth and gum problems. When a person takes care of themselves they will have more energy, be less thirsty, urinate less often, heal better, and have few skin and bladder infections. Therefore, monitoring the disease and taking the advice from a doctor is the best way to go.

Chapter 2 – Type One and Type Two Diabetes

Type 1 Diabetes

Knowing which type of diabetes that has been diagnosed will help an individual figure out their meal plan, exercise plan, and which types of medications they may have to take to regulate their glucose levels. There are three different types of diabetes. The most severe type of diabetes is Type 1. Type 2 is the next most severe, and gestational is the least severe.

Type 1 diabetes is the most severe of the three types because it is incurable and can be caused by a lot of different factors. People who have had pancreatic surgery or cystic fibrosis may develop secondary diabetes because the beta cells that carry the insulin are being destroyed. This does not allow the body to get nutrients and sugar to the other cells of the body because the insulin is no longer there to convert the sugar. People with this type of diabetes must take insulin every day to survive.

Type 1 diabetes that has gone untreated may cause severe health conditions that may even lead to death. Some of these conditions include dehydration, weight loss, diabetic ketoacidosis, and damage to the body due to lack of nutrients to the cells. Dehydration is caused by the body trying to flush the extra glucose out through the body, which is carried out with urine. Increased urination will cause dehydration. Weight loss is caused by the dehydration because calories are also expelled through the urine. People with Type 1 diabetes will feel hungry and eat more but continue to lose weight.

Diabetic ketoacidosis is a complex process where the cells are starved of energy and the body begins to break down fat cells to attempt reversing this starvation. When the fat breaks down, acidic chemicals known as ketones are released into the bloodstream. These ketones build up in the blood, and the liver continues to release sugar in an attempt to balance everything out. Because the body is unable to use these sugars, it continues to build up in the bloodstream and eventually causes high sugar, dehydration, and acidic buildup known as ketoacidosis. This complication can be life-threatening if it's not dealt with immediately.

Although this complication is rare for people who have had the disease less than fifteen years, it occurs in eighty percent of adults who have had the disease for longer than that timeframe. Retinopathy is the loss of vision in one or both eyes, but it is preventable. Patients must management their blood pressure, regulate their blood fats like cholesterol and triglycerides, and need to keep their insulin levels regulated. Fortunately, complete vision loss can be avoided for most people.

The cause of Type 1 diabetes is still unknown, but it obvious to scientists and doctors that the susceptibility is hereditary. However, they have identified that an environmental trigger plays a role in causing diabetes, and they've narrowed it down to either being a toxin or a virus. This environmental trigger causes the immune system to attack the beta cells of the pancreas, thus destroying them to the point where they can no longer function. There are markers to the destruction known as autoantibodies, which can be seen in eighty-five to ninety percent of the people with the condition. Because Type 1 diabetes is an autoimmune disease, other autoimmune diseases may occur and should be looked out for.

Symptoms that may hint at an emergency with Type 1 diabetes include shaking and confusion, rapid breathing, fruity smell on the breath, abdominal pain, and loss of consciousness. All of these symptoms should be addressed with a doctor immediately or an emergency healthcare responder. They can be signs of glucose levels in the blood being dangerously high or low.

Type 2 Diabetes

Type 2 diabetes was known as non-insulin-dependent diabetes. It is the most common form and affects ninety to ninety-five percent of Americans with diabetes. Unlike people who have Type 1 diabetes, people with Type 2 diabetes make insulin, but their pancreas is not making enough or their body cannot use the insulin properly. The same thing occurs with people who have Type 2 diabetes as it does with people who have Type 1, the body is unable to get imperative nutrients to the other cells and they begin to starve.

Type 2 diabetes may be more common than Type 1, but there is less known about it than its more dangerous counterpart. It runs in families and may be caused by some of the same environmental factors, although it is more commonly associated with people who are overweight. People who are more at risk for developing Type 2 diabetes are men and women who are over the age of forty-five, obese or overweight, had gestational diabetes, have family members who have Type 2 diabetes, had prediabetes, low HDL cholesterol or high triglycerides, have high blood pressure, are members of the African-American, Latino, Native American, Asian American or Pacific Islanders, and have a low activity level.

People with Type 2 diabetes may experience many of the complications of Type 1 diabetes such as damage to the body over time, dehydration, and diabetic coma. Damage to the body may include nerve damage, small blood vessels of the eyes, kidneys, and heart that may lead to atherosclerosis, which is a hardening of the arteries that may cause heart attack and stroke. Dehydration is caused by buildup of sugar in the blood that causes an increase in urination. Once this dehydration reaches a certain point, whether because the diabetic person has too much sugar or has become dehydrated from illness, they could fall into a diabetic coma. A diabetic coma is a serious, life-threatening and event and the person will need medical attention immediately.

The same tests will be run to determine if a person has Type 2 diabetes and the same complications can arise. The person will go through two tests that measure the glucose levels in the blood. They may develop kidney problems, heart complications, poor circulation that leads to nerve damage, and retinopathy.

Type 2 diabetes is treated like Type 1 diabetes except that people diagnosed with this less threatening version of diabetes do not need to take insulin permanently.

Chapter 3 – Gestational Diabetes and Prediabetes

Gestational Diabetes

A condition characterized by high blood sugar levels first recognized during pregnancy, gestational diabetes occurred in about four percent of pregnant women. Most women have a degree of weakened glucose intolerance because of hormonal changes during pregnancy. Their blood sugar may be higher than normal, but it's not high enough to have diabetes. Gestational diabetes usually happens in the third trimester.

The cause of gestational diabetes is very clear. The placenta produces hormones in order to make the mother's body produce enough nutrients for the fetus. Sometimes these hormones lead to impaired glucose intolerance, which the body then creates more insulin to get the glucose into the mother's cells so she can use them for energy. Occasionally, the mother's pancreas does not react accordingly and cannot produce enough insulin to take care of the extra glucose, thus resulting in gestational diabetes.

There are certain factors that increase the risk of having gestational diabetes. A woman who is overweight before she is pregnant, twenty percent or more over the ideal body weight, may develop gestational diabetes and perhaps Type 2 diabetes if she does not get her weight under control after having the baby. Other risk factors include: previously giving birth to a baby over nine pounds, a previous stillborn, too much amniotic fluid, and an impaired glucose tolerance. However, numerous women develop gestational diabetes and do not have any of these known risk factors.

Women who are at high risk for developing gestational diabetes should be screened as early as possible while pregnant in order to make sure the fetus has the best chance possible. Women without risk are screened between the twenty-fourth and twenty-eighth weeks of pregnancy. The normal test is an oral glucose tolerance test. It involves drinking a liquid with fifty grams of sugar in it quickly. The body will absorb the sugar and it will cause the sugar levels to rise within an hour. The sample will be taken from a vein and the blood test will tell the doctors if the sugar solution was processed. If the sugar level is greater than one hundred and forty milligrams per deciliter, then the results are abnormal.

If the oral glucose tolerance test comes back abnormal, the woman will take another test after fasting for several hours in order to confirm. Women who come back normal will be tested at the twenty-four to twenty-eight week mark to make sure. It is imperative to have this test done in order to know how to effectively treat the illness in order to keep the fetus healthy.

Unfortunately, women who do not have this test performed who are at risk for developing gestational diabetes risk their baby's life. Gestational diabetes can cause birth defects that affect the major organs such as the brain and heart, which can lead to a miscarriage. Later on in the pregnancy, it can cause a baby to have too much nutrition and grow too quickly, thus endangering the mother and child during labor. An emergency caesarean may need to be performed. In addition, the child is still at risk of its blood sugar levels dropping too low after it's born because it has been detached from the mother, who was supplying vast amounts of glucose in the blood. All of these risks are life threatening to the child and should be taken seriously.

Thankfully, there are ways to manage gestational diabetes. These ways include monitoring blood sugar levels before breakfast, two hours after meals, and in the evening. The urine will be monitored for ketones, and the woman must follow dietary guidelines laid out by her doctor. Calorie distribution throughout the day is important. Some women are allowed to exercise after they've been given a diagnosis, and are encouraged to monitor their weight gain. Insulin is the only drug that can be taken by diabetic, pregnant women at this time. And lastly, women should monitor their blood pressure to make sure it's not too high.

Knowing when to eat and what to eat can become overwhelming, but it's not as difficult as it may seem. Women with gestational diabetes should eat three meals a day and snacks in between. They cannot skip a meal or snack and must keep their carbohydrates between forty and forty-five percent of their total calorie intake at breakfast. A snack before bed should consist of fifteen to thirty grams of carbohydrates. Women with morning sickness should eat one to two servings of crackers, pretzels, or cereal before they get out of bed. All pregnant women should consume twenty to thirty-five grams of fiber daily, and can obtain these foods from whole grain breads, pasta, cereals, fruits, rice, and vegetables. Along with fiber, women should consume eight cups of liquid a day. All women should take prenatal vitamins to ensure their child is getting the best nutrition possible.

Not everything is over after the delivery. Doctors will immediately test a baby's glucose levels and give them a sugar solution through intravenous means or orally in order to get the baby's glucose readings to the right level. The mother will be tested immediately to make sure she hadn't experienced a drop in blood sugar levels, and she will need to be tested six to twelve weeks after delivery to ensure her diabetes has disappeared. However, women who have experienced gestational diabetes should be tested periodically by their doctors because they have a sixty percent chance of developing diabetes later on in life.

If a woman decides to become pregnant again after having gestational diabetes, she has a forty to fifty percent chance of developing the disease again. Thus, all women should be tested for gestational diabetes while pregnant. It may not be the easiest illness to monitor during pregnancy, but it will be worth it in the end.

Prediabetes

Seventy nine million people over the age of twenty in the United States alone are estimated to have prediabetes. This condition is determined through a glucose test that comes back above the normal range, but it's not high enough to be diagnosed as Type 2 diabetes. Eventually, people diagnosed with prediabetes will develop diabetes if they do not treat the condition early on. More and more doctors are recognizing that they should screen patients for glucose levels to make sure they are not at risk for developing diabetes.

People who are at risk for developing prediabetes have a family history of diabetes. Women who have had gestational diabetes or had a baby that weighed more than nine pounds are at risk. In addition, women who have polycystic ovary syndrome are at risk for developing prediabetes that will turn into type 2 diabetes. People who are overweight or obese, especially those who have excess belly fat, are at risk. Older people, especially those with high cholesterol, triglycerides, low HDL, and high LDL, are at risk for developing prediabetes. Lastly, people who do not exercise enough daily are at risk.

Treating prediabetes will eradicate the problem and lower a person's risk for a positive diabetic test later on in life. People who have been diagnosed with prediabetes should eat a heart healthy diet and lose five to ten percent of their overall weight. Exercising for thirty minutes a day, five days a week can significantly lower risk. People who smoke should quit and people with high blood pressure and cholesterol should effectively treat it.

Chapter 4 – Foods to Avoid

Choosing the right foods and the right amounts while managing diabetes can be overwhelming at first; therefore, this section will be broken down into the different types of foods, and which ones are healthy in that category to consume. Remember, each person is different and how they react to these different types of food will be on an individual basis. That is why it's appropriate to start out slow and test often to see how the individual is reacting to the different types of foods.

Fats

There are two different types of fats when it comes to food fats. There are unhealthy fats and there are healthy fats. Fats categorized as unhealthy include saturated, trans and cholesterol. Healthy fats include monounsaturated, polyunsaturated, and omega-3 fatty acids.

For people with diabetes, saturated fat is even worse than people who are not diagnosed with the disease. Saturated fat raises a person's cholesterol levels in their bloodstream, which puts them at a higher risk for heart attack and stroke. People who have been diagnosed with diabetes are already at a higher risk; therefore, they do not want to double that risk. The goal is to consume less than ten percent of the daily diet worth of saturated fat, which is twenty grams or less for the average person.

Foods that are high in saturated fat include:

- Fatback and salt pork
- High-fat meats (regular ground beef, bologna, hot dogs, sausage, bacon, spareribs)
- Lard

* Full-fat cheese

* Ice Cream

* Whole Milk

* 2% Milk

* Sour Cream

* Butter

* Cream sauces

* Gravy with meat drippings

* Chocolate

* Palm Oil

* Kernel Oil

* Coconut

* Coconut Oil

* Poultry Skin

Trans-fat also increases the cholesterol in the bloodstream. It's worse than saturated fat for the heart, so it's even more advisable to avoid than most other fats. Trans-fat is created when liquid oil is made into a solid fat through the process of hydrogenation. They are listed on all food labels, but the food must contain more than 0.5 grams of trans-fat to be listed on the label; otherwise, the company can put 0 grams on the label. Therefore, a person avoiding this type of fat should look at the ingredients list. If it contains anything that says hydrogenated or partially hydrogenated oil, it has trans-fat in it.

Foods that contain trans-fat include:

* French Fries or other fast food items

* Processed snacks such as crackers and chips

- Baked goods such as muffins, cookies, and cakes,

- Stick margarines and shortening

Cholesterol is a naturally occurring substance in the bloodstream. Most of it is made from the body itself, but some of it comes from foods a person consumes. All animal foods are sources of dietary cholesterol. Food companies are required to put cholesterol on the label if the food contains any amounts of it. It's a good idea to keep cholesterol consumption at or around three hundred milligrams per day.

Foods that have cholesterol include:

- Whole or 2% milk, cream, ice cream, full-fat cheese

- Egg yolks

- Liver and organ meats

- Meat and Poultry skin

Alcohol

People with severe diabetes should avoid alcohol, but people with less severe cases such as type 2 diabetes or prediabetes can consume alcohol. It is recommended they consume it with food and no more than the recommended amount for normal people: no more than one drink daily for women and no more than two for men. A drink consists of a twelve ounce beer, five ounces of wine, or one and a half ounces of distilled spirits.

Beverages

Sugary drinks are, of course, a no-no. These may include things such as soda, fruit juice, energy drinks, sweet tea, and fruit punch. Just one drink can be the equivalent to ten teaspoons of sugar, which is highly detrimental to a person's blood glucose levels.

Chapter 5 – Foods to Eat

Fats

Monounsaturated fat is considered a healthy fat, but there are guidelines. A lot of foods that contain monounsaturated fat also include bad fats; therefore, moderation is still important. These are known as good fats because they lower the LDL or bad cholesterol in the bloodstream.

Sources of these fats include:

- Avocados
- Sesame Seeds
- Peanut butter and oil
- Nuts
- Canola oil
- Olive oil and olives

Polyunsaturated fats work just like monounsaturated fats in the diet. They lower the bad cholesterol in the bloodstream. Foods that include polyunsaturated fats are:

- Cottonseed oil
- Safflower oil
- Corn oil
- Soybean oil
- Sunflower oil

- Walnuts
- Sunflower or pumpkin seeds
- Walnuts
- Soft (tub) margarine
- Mayonnaise
- Salad dressings

The final, healthy fats are omega-3 fatty acids. These help prevent clogging of the arteries and one of the highest foods with these in it is fish. The American Diabetes Association recommends everyone consumes fish at least two to three times weekly.

Some foods rich in omega-3 fatty acids are:

- Mackerel
- Herring
- Albacore tuna
- Rainbow trout
- Salmon
- Sardines
- Tofu
- Soybean products
- Flaxseed and flaxseed oil
- Walnuts
- Canola oil

<u>***Non-Starchy Vegetables***</u>

People with diabetes should fill up on these vegetables because they do not raise blood sugar levels. If a person who is diabetic is feeling hungry, but they know their glucose levels are too high, they can still munch on several foods that fall into this category. People with and without diabetes should consume anywhere from three to five servings of vegetables daily as a minimum. These vegetables contain high amounts of nutrients and vitamins; therefore, people with diabetes will not lack nutrition because they cannot eat as much as other people.

Non-starchy vegetables include:

- Amaranth
- Artichoke
- Asparagus
- Baby Corn
- Beans
- Bamboo Shoots
- Beets
- Brussels sprouts
- Cabbage
- Carrots
- Celery
- Cauliflower
- Chayote
- Coleslaw
- Cucumber

- Eggplant
- Greens (Collard, Kale, Mustard, Turnips)
- Jicama
- Kohlrabi
- Mushrooms
- Onions
- Pea pods
- Okra
- Peppers
- Radishes
- Salad greens
- Rutabaga
- Tomatoes
- Turnips
- Water chestnuts
- Yardlong beans

Grains and Starchy Vegetables

There is a large debate on whether or not grains help or hinder people who are trying to lose weight and people diagnosed with diabetes. There is one thing that seems to be a consensus: when choosing grains, always choose whole grains. Cut out the processed foods that contain grains and put in the ones that are made from healthier grains such as:

- Whole wheat flour
- Whole oats/oatmeal

* Bulgur

* Whole grain corn/corn meal

* Brown rice

* Popcorn

* Whole rye

* Whole grain barley

* Wild rice

* Whole faro

* Buckwheat

* Triticale

* Millet

* Quinoa

* Sorghum

Starchy vegetables are something that should be consumed in moderation unless they are some of the following:

* Plantain
* Parsnip
* Potato
* Pumpkin
* Corn
* Green peas
* Acorn squash
* Butternut squash
* Dred beans
* Lentils

- Dried peas

- Vegetarian baked beans

- Fat-free refried beans

Protein

Most sources of protein do not raise glucose levels; therefore, consuming them at will is not detrimental. The best choices of protein are plant-based, fish, seafood, chicken, cheese, and eggs. Red meat may have fat in it that can raise glucose levels.

For plant-based protein, try these:

- Beans

- Hummus

- Peas

- Edamame

- Soy nuts

- Lentils

- Tempeh

- Vegetarian meat substitutes

For fish and seafood, try these:

- Albacore tuna

- Mackerel

- Herring

- Rainbow trout
- Sardines
- Salmon
- Catfish
- Cod
- Flounder
- Haddock
- Orange roughy
- Tilapia
- Clams
- Crab
- Lobster
- Scallops
- Shrimp
- Oysters

For poultry, try these:

- Chicken
- Turkey
- Cornish hen

For Cheese and Eggs:

- Reduced-fat cheese
- Cottage cheese
- Egg whites

- Egg substitutes

For game items, try these:

- Buffalo
- Rabbit
- Venison
- Ostrich
- Dove
- Duck
- Goose
- Pheasant (no skin)

There are some red meats that are okay to consume, but they should be the leanest options such as:

- Beef trimmed of fat (chuck, rib, rump roast, sirloin, cubed, flank, porterhouse, T-bone steak, tenderloin)
- Beef jerky
- Lamb
- Organ meats
- Veal
- Pork

Beverages

There are alternatives to water! Not everyone with diabetes must consume only water, which might be boring after a while. While there are a few beverages that must be avoided, there are several that can be consumed.

These beverages include:

- Hot or cold black, green, and herbal teas that are unsweetened
- Sparkling water
- Water infused with cucumbers, strawberries, or fresh mint
- Diet drinks such as diet soda or tea
- Low calorie drink mixes
- Low-fat milk
- 100% juice with no added sweeteners
- Milk
- Soy milk
- Rice milk
- Almond milk

Fruits

Almost all fruits are safe for diabetic people to eat. In fact, they're a great source of vitamins and fiber. When choosing canned fruit, it should be processed in natural juices. The following is a list of common fruit that is safe for diabetics:

- Apples
- Apricots
- Banana

- Applesauce
- Blackberries
- Blueberries
- Cantaloupe
- Dates
- Cherries
- Dried fruit
- Fruit cocktail
- Figs
- Grapes
- Grapefruit
- Kiwi
- Honeydew melon
- Nectarine
- Mango
- Orange
- Papaya
- Plums
- Peaches
- Pears
- Raspberries
- Tangerines
- Strawberries
- Watermelon

Chapter 6 – Coping with Diabetes

There are numerous different ways to cope with diabetes. The American Diabetes Association recommends that a person with diabetes have someone who is a close family member, friend, or even a professional that they can talk to whenever they need to about the stress of handling diabetes. Because this disease is a full-time complication that will most likely never go away, it can be extremely stressful. It's not as simple as monitoring what a person eats or their blood sugar occasionally, it's about keeping on top of their blood sugar constantly so that they do not have any other complications.

People who have been diagnosed with diabetes should speak with someone who will listen when they are having trouble. They can join a support group that has a diabetes educator, or even create their own discussion group to talk about important matters. The best thing to do is to keep busy and stop allowing the disease to run their life. Starting a hobby such as taking a dance class or volunteering will help. If reading or getting a massage will help them relax, they should make sure to do it more often. Most importantly, diabetic people should not hide from their friends and family. They need that support group around them to cope with the frightening diagnosis.

If a diabetic person is experiencing fear, then they should take care of themselves first and find a way to deal with their fear in a healthy manner. Understanding the risks and long-term health problems will help a diabetic understand the future and come to terms with how their life is going to be. Anyone diagnosed with this disease should seek out as much information as they can in order to understand the disease fully.

Depression is an unfortunate, common complication with diabetes. Taking care of the illness can be complex, demanding, and very frustrating. Talking to a professional will always help with this, and there is no shame in needing the advice of someone well educated with the disease. Some symptoms of this secondary illness are anxiety, loss of interest in activities or trouble falling asleep.

It is completely understandable that someone with this diagnosis would feel hopeless and depressed.

The four ways to cope with this disease are to eat healthily, be active, remember the medication, and keep track of food intake and glucose levels. Once these four, basic cornerstones of coping with diabetes have been meant, the patient will feel much better and much more in control of their own life.

Chapter 7 – Medical Management

To first understand medical management of diabetes, it is best to know what the definition of diabetes is and what type a person has. Diabetes is the decreased or lack of production of insulin in the body. Type one diabetes occurs when the body no longer has the ability to produce any type of insulin. Type two diabetes occurs when the body is able to produce insulin, but it's not enough to keep up with the demands of the individual. Therefore, type one diabetics must have insulin daily to keep their blood sugar levels in check while type two diabetics may or may not need insulin. Type two diabetics might be able to survive on oral medication to manage their diabetes, or they may rely on diet and exercise alone to get their diabetes under control. Both of these methods will be explained.

Insulin

This naturally occurring hormone that is secreted by the pancreas is the culprit of diabetes. It is the lack of this hormone in the body that causes a person to go into diabetic shock. People with type one diabetes are always prescribed insulin to keep their glucose levels maintained. Some people with type two diabetes are prescribed insulin for a short period of time or low doses to maintain their glucose levels. There are more than twenty different types of insulin sold in the United States alone, and they all differ in how they're made, how they work, and their cost.

There are four main different types of insulin. These include rapid-acting, regular, intermediate, and long-acting. For people who have difficulty mixing their insulin, premixed prescriptions are available. The most common strength of insulin available is U-100, and all insulin available in the United States is manufactured by a laboratory. However, sometimes doctors can have insulin made from animals imported for their patients.

Rapid-acting insulin will begin to work fifteen minutes after the injection, and it peaks within an hour. The medication continues to work for two to four hours after the injection. Regular insulin reaches the bloodstream thirty minutes after it's injected and peaks two to three hours after injection. It is effective for three to six hours. Intermediate insulin reaches the bloodstream two to four hours after injection and peaks at four to twelve hours later. It is effective anywhere from twelve to eighteen hours. Finally, long-acting insulin reaches the bloodstream several hours after it is injected and will keep glucose levels even over a twenty-four hour period. It is best to know which type of insulin a person has in order to make sure they are obtaining the correct dose.

Depending upon the type of diabetes a person has, their dosage will and how many times they inject during the day will be different. Normally, people will type one diabetes will start with two injections a day with two different types of insulin, and then they will progress to three or four injections of different types daily. Scientific studies show these dosage amounts prolong a person's quality of life and prevent or delay eye, kidney, and nerve damage caused by the disease.

People with type two diabetes may need one injection of insulin a day without diabetic oral medications. Usually, these injections are taken in the evening along with their medication if they need anything else. Some people with type two diabetes may become resistant to the one injection daily and may need to uptake their injections by two or three a day. In rare cases, they may need to go to four injections per day. It all depends upon the individual and their personal circumstances.

Oral Medications

People with type one diabetes are not able to manage their disease with just oral medication, they must take insulin. When a person is able to use only oral medications to manage their diabetes, that person should pair it with exercise and diet therapy. Pills do not work for everyone, and while some people find that their glucose levels decrease, they do not decrease to the appropriate levels.

There are several different types of oral medications used for diabetes that have been approved by the FDA and are used by doctors. These medications have been tested and proven effective using both animal and human trials. Therefore, they are safe when prescribed by a doctor. These drugs include sulfonylureas, biguanides, meglitinides, thiazolidinediones, SGLT2 Inhibitors, DPP-4 Inhibitors, Alpha-glucosidase inhibitors, and Bile Acid Sequestrants.

There are three different types of sulfonylureas: first-generation, second-generation, and third-generation. All three of them have similar effects on glucose levels, but their side effects differ and their reactions with other drugs are different. Therefore, it is imperative to make sure to tell the doctor what other medications are being taken before beginning a sulfonylureas regiment. This medication works by stimulating the beta cells in the pancreas to release more insulin.

Biguanides are usually taken two times a day and help lower glucose levels by decreasing the amount of glucose produced by the liver. In addition, they make muscle tissue more sensitive to insulin so the glucose can be absorbed. A side effect of this medication may be diarrhea, but taking the drug with food can improve this.

Meglitinides are like sulfonylureas because they stimulate the beta cells to release insulin. Doctors recommend they be taken before the three, main meals a day and do not usually prescribe them with sulfonylureas because they can cause hypoglycemia when taken in excess. Alcohol and some diabetic medications do not mix because they cause vomiting, flushing or sickness, and meglitinides are one of the medications not safe to be taken with alcohol.

There is debate about the drugs within the thiazolidinediones category. One of them, Rezulin, was removed from the market because a few people experienced liver complications. This group of drugs reduces glucose from the liver and helps bond insulin with muscle and fat. The other two drugs, rosiglitazone and pioglitazone do not appear to have the same issues as Rezulin, but both drugs should be taken with caution as they have shown to increase the risk for heart attacks in some individuals.

Inhibitors are a specific type of drug that try to block certain nutrients from being absorbed in the body. DPP-4 inhibitors prevent the breakdown of GLP-1 in the body. SGLT2 inhibitors work to block the action of the kidneys absorbing glucose so that it may be eliminated in the urine. Alpha-glucosidase inhibitors block the breakdown of starches in the bloodstream, and they slow the breakdown of sugars. All of these medications should be taken with a meal.

Bile acid Sequestrants are actually used to lower cholesterol in patients with high LDL levels. It has been shown to help patients with diabetes by lowering blood glucose levels, too. It binds the bile acids in the digestive tract, and the body uses cholesterol to substitute the bile acids. Thus, the cholesterol is eliminated from the body naturally.

While all of these medications are viable remedies to help manage diabetes, they may interact with each other and different medications. Sulfonylureas and meglitinides can cause hypoglycemia, metformin may cause hypoglycemia if taken with insulin, and acarbose or meglitol may cause hypoglycemia if taken with other diabetic medications. It is important to talk with a doctor about all medications, even over the counter ones, being taken.

Chapter 8 – Diet Management

People who have been diagnosed with type two diabetes have the opportunity to lower their disease level or eliminate it with diet management. Even people with type one diabetes will benefit from losing weight if they are overweight, and watching what they eat will help keep their blood glucose levels in check. Women who want to lose weight should remember that a healthy waist circumference is thirty-five inches or less, and a man's healthy waist circumference is forty inches or less.

There are several myths associated with diabetes when it comes to eating. The first myth is that diabetics must avoid sugar completely. Dessert should be planned accordingly and combined with a healthy meal plan or exercise. The second myth is that a high-protein diet is best. The truth is that eating too much protein may increase the risk for diabetes because it can cause insulin resistance. A healthy, balanced diet is the best way to go.

Another myth is that diabetics must cut back significantly on their carb intake. The truth is that diabetics must eat a balanced diet, and this means carbs must be consumed at a healthy level. Whole grain carbs are the best and they're an excellent source of fiber, which is digested slowly and helps keep blood sugar levels even. The fourth myth is that diabetics cannot eat normally and must eat a special diabetic meal plan. The truth is that healthy eating is universal, and there are no special, diabetic foods that will make everything better. Eating in moderation is key, and substitution is an excellent way to enjoy foods while eating out with family and friends.

For example, substituting sweet potatoes for white potatoes or brown rice for white rice are both great choices. Try using whole-wheat breads and pastas instead of white. Eat breakfast cereal that is high in fiber instead of loaded with sugar. Even ordering peas or leafy greens instead of corn when eating out will help. Some more foods that are safe to eat are:

- Fruits (apples, pears, peaches, berries, bananas, mangoes, and papayas)

- Beans

- Millet

- Fish

- Skinless Chicken

- Olive Oil

- Nuts

- Avocados

- Many More!

It is important to remember to have three meals a day and only one to two snacks. Most diabetics make the mistake of skipping breakfast, which is an important meal for any person during the day. In addition, make sure to eat slowly and train the brain on how to realize when the stomach is full. Try eating for ten minutes and then stopping for five. Below are some more powerful foods that help people with diabetes.

When it comes to breakfast, oatmeal is an excellent choice for people with diabetes and people who are looking to eat healthy in general. It is important to remember not to get the sweetened kind of oatmeal. Oatmeal acts like a cleaner because it has so much fiber in it, which helps control blood sugar levels. It also helps people feel fuller, longer.

Broccoli, spinach, and green beans are great sources of fiber and they're low in carbohydrates. They're part of a group known as non-starchy vegetables. Unlike their bad cousin, starch vegetables such as potatoes, peas, corn, winter squash, and lima beans, non-starchy vegetables do not have to be monitored as much when they're eaten. Thus, people can fill up on these vegetables without feeling guilty.

When the craving for a cookie or candy comes along, strawberries are an excellent substitute. A cup of strawberries is a healthy snack that will not raise blood sugar levels too high and they're low in calories and carbohydrates. The longer people stay full, the more weight they will lose, and strawberries help curb those pesky cravings.

Meat is a source of chromium, which is a mineral that helps insulin function and also helps the body metabolize carbohydrates. There are specific meats that are better at doing this than others. Those meats include salmon, lean cuts, and skinless chicken breast.

Some people do not like the option of drinking diet sodas in lieu of regular soda because there are some health complications that go along with diet soda and it has been proven to cause weight gain. There is a healthy alternative that will eliminate the desire for something fizzy. Sparkling water either plain or flavored with a squeeze of lemon or lime juice is an excellent alternative. Grocery stores carry many different varieties with unique flavors such as apple-pear, bananas, tangerine, and grapefruit.

When it comes to dieting with diabetes, remembering to keep to portion sizes is imperative. However, there are many excellent choices and eating out does not have to become an exhausting event. Remembering to stick with lean meats, non-starchy vegetables, and a small dessert are all easy things to recall.

Chapter 9 – Herbal Management

There are some skeptics out there who believe herbal remedies are a crock, but some of them have been proven to work with scientific studies. Many of them seem odd or even outrageous, but they work with people who have type 2 diabetes. People with type 1 diabetes cannot supplement or replace their insulin with herbal remedies.

Some common herbal remedy management options are as follows:

Agaricus Mushroom

The Agaricus mushroom is a fungus that originated in Brazil, but it is now grown in Japan, China, and Brazil for commercial resale. The extract taken from the plant is used as a remedy for cancer, type 2 diabetes, high cholesterol, artery hardening, liver disease, digestive disorders, and bloodstream disorders. When it comes to diabetes, the Agaricus mushroom contains some chemicals that help the body use insulin and decreases insulin resistance in people who use it.

Beer

It seems odd, but the alcohol drink known as beer is used in small amounts for various reasons. Some of these reasons include heart failure, heart attack, stroke, and hardening of the arteries. All of these complications can be experienced by people with type one and two diabetes; therefore, they use beer to decrease their risk of these complications. It works by increasing HDL cholesterol or good cholesterol in the bloodstream.

Blond psyllium

Blond psyllium, or commercially known as Metamucil, is the seed and husk of the seed used as a laxative or for softening stool. The husk of the seed absorbs water and forms a large mass. When this happens in people with constipation, a common side-effect of people with diabetes, the mass stimulates the bowel to move. People with diarrhea will experience a slowdown of bowel movements.

Chromium

Chromium should not be used without the care of a doctor. Too low doses can cause hypoglycemia, especially when it is taken with prescription medications. Too high of a dose can cause kidney damage. It is an essential trace element that is used to metabolize carbohydrates, which means it may have some effects at helping weight loss and keeping glucose levels in check.

Vitamin B1

People diagnosed with diabetes are also diagnosed as being thiamine deficient. Low levels of this B vitamin can cause heart disease and blood vessel damage. It is a water-soluble vitamin and has a hard time being absorbed by cells. Benfotiamine is a supplement form of thiamine and can more easily penetrate cell membranes. This vitamin may be able to prevent diabetic complications.

Alpha-Lipoic Acid

Alpha-Lipoic Acid or ALA should be taken with a doctor's observations as it can cause hypoglycemia in some patients. However, studies have shown that it has the potential to lower blood sugar levels, decrease insulin resistance, and reduce oxidative stress on cells. It is a very strong antioxidant.

Bitter Melon

Bitter melon appears to show promise when it comes to animal and lab studies, but there is no conclusive data. It has a modest effect on lowering blood sugar levels, but it is not as effective as metformin. However, for people who are prediabetic and people who have a mild case of diabetes, bitter melon may be effective.

Fenugreek

The fenugreek plant is used for numerous conditions, and the seeds are used to make medication. The seeds slow the absorption of sugars and stimulate insulin production. For people with diabetes, the effects lower blood sugar levels.

Flaxseed

Both the seed and oil from the Linum usitatissimum plant are used to make medication. This pertains to medication made from the seed. It is used for numerous gastrointestinal complications such as diarrhea, inflammation, colon damage, constipation, and irritable bowel syndrome. It is also used for people with diabetes because it is an excellent source of fiber and omega-3 fatty acids. It helps people with type two diabetes who are trying to lose weight feel fuller so that they may eat less.

Ginseng

American ginseng is a herb where the root is used to make the medication. It is excellent for stress and boosting the immune system, and is a general stimulant. The American version of ginseng contains a chemical that affects insulin levels in the body and lowers blood sugar. Chemicals known as polysaccharides are what affect the immune system.

Glucomannan

Glucomannan may seem like an odd choice because it is actually a sugar made from the root of the konjac plant. It comes in powders, capsules and tablets and is commonly used for constipation and weight loss. It works in the intestines and stomach by absorbing water to form a sort of plug. This slows the absorption of cholesterol and sugar from the stomach, which then helps control sugar levels.

Green Tea

Green tea is generally considered safe for people with diabetes. However, it should be the unsweetened kind, not sweetened. It contains polyphenols which are an antioxidant, and it contains epigallocatechin gallate, which is known to have health benefits such as improving insulin activity, glucose control, and lowering cardiovascular disease risk.

Guar Gum

Guar gum is a fiber derived from the seed of the plant that helps the digestive tract. It can decrease the levels of cholesterol and glucose absorbed in the intestines, thus lowering glucose levels. It expands in the intestines and is currently being studied as a weight loss supplement because the expansion causes a sense of fullness.

Resveratrol

A chemical found in grapes and wine, resveratrol has been shown to prevent high blood sugar. It also reduces oxidative stress, thus helping the cells function properly. While this chemical has been used in animal studies and it's been successful, human studies have not been conducted.

Soy

Soy, derived from the soybean plant, are processed into a protein. It comes in many forms such as powder, milk, and fiber. It is used for high cholesterol, blood pressure, and prevents heart disease. When used for type two diabetes, soy helps lower blood glucose levels.

White Mulberry

An herbal supplement that is derived from the leaves, white mulberry is effective in treating type two diabetes. It is also used to treat cholesterol levels, blood pressure, the common cold, muscle and joint pains, constipation, dizziness, hair loss, ringing in the ears, and premature graying. When utilized for diabetic purposes, white mulberry has some properties of other, commercial drugs used. It slows the breakdown of sugars in the stomach and helps keep blood sugar levels in a healthy range.

Magnesium

Magnesium is an essential nutrient in the human body. It will help regulate blood pressure and insulin sensitivity. A diet high in this nutrient will reduce the risk of diabetes and lower rates of insulin resistance.

Chapter 10 – Stress Management

Stress is a very common side-effect of diabetes because people diagnosed with the disease do not know how to manage their daily lives with this newfound obstacle. While it may not seem like a big deal when compared to the disease of diabetes, stress can cause severe complications. And let's face it, no one needs added stress in their lives.

The clinical definition of stress is a physical or mental reaction to the apparent danger. Disease that seem uncontrollable or require some sort of change is perceived as a threat by the human mind. Once the body and mind have sensed a threat, the fight or flight mode kicks in. This informs the body it needs to increase several hormones within the body that are secreted by a few key areas of the brain and glands. This complex occurrence can cause an increase in blood glucose levels, impair thinking, incite negative emotions, and create poor eating habits.

Whether a person who is diabetic or not experiences stress over a long period of time, it will be harmful due to wear and tear caused in the body. Prolonged stress can affect the immune system, digestive tract, kidneys, and reproductive organs. When all of these organs work harder than they need to for a prolonged amount of time, people begin to develop secondary illnesses. Illnesses already present will get worse. In some cases, this chronic stress can develop into depression.

There are numerous symptoms when it comes to stress. These symptoms can be broken down into four groups: physical, emotional, cognitive, and behavioral. Seeing any or all of these symptoms in either one's self or someone they know is a sure sign that a person needs to consult a physician about what they are feeling.

The physical symptoms of stress may include the following:

- Hands shaking

- Palpitations

- Heartburn or indigestion

- Shortness of breath

- Upset stomach

- Diarrhea

- Constipation

- Nausea

- Muscle tension

- Low energy

- Tingling of fingers or around mouth

- Sweating

- Grinding of the teeth

- Difficulty swallowing

- Ringing in the ears

- Cold hands and feet

- Low or no sexual desire

- Pain

- Aches

- Insomnia

- Frequent colds or infections

Emotional symptoms of stress might include:

- Irrational nervousness

- Moodiness

- Frustration

- Feeling of being overwhelmed

- Lonely

- Feeling worthless

- Easily agitated

- Avoidance of others

- Low self-esteem

- Unable to relax

- Self-conscious

Cognitive symptoms of stress might include:

- Forgetfulness

- Racing thoughts

- Poor judgment

- Worrying

- Behavior symptoms may include:

- Changes in appetite

- Procrastination

- Loss of interest in hobbies and work

- Abuse of alcohol, drugs, or cigarettes

- Nail biting, pacing, fidgeting

Managing stress may seem like it's a lost cause or that there is no hope, but there is. Stress is merely a physical reaction to an outside force put on the person, and by managing the disease of diabetes, the stress will start to dissipate. In the meantime, there are several ways to reduce stress in a diabetic person's life or any person's life.

The first thing to remember is keeping a positive attitude. Things may seem as if they are going wrong, and it's easier to see the bad rather than the good when stressed. Finding something that is good in each part of a person's life such as work, friends, family, and health are a good way to start. This will help a person change their mindset and think about the positive rather than the negative.

People feeling stress need to remember to be kind to themselves. It's okay to say 'no' to something that makes them feel uncomfortable or that stretches their time too thin. Expecting too much out of themselves is a common side-effect of being too stressed out. Diabetics must learn to put themselves ahead of others when it comes to what they do with their time, and they must remember that they are human. It is okay to be conscious of what they need.

Acceptance is something that is difficult for most people. Sometimes things that cause stress can be eliminated, but other times they are unavoidable. Remember to ask if the situation will be important years from the time when it happens, whether or not there is any control over it, and if it can be changed. If it can be changed, then by all means, change it. But if it cannot, learn how to let go of the stress and move on.

Sometimes, moving on from a stressor is more difficult than it seems and professional help may be needed. Talking to a professional about stress is never something to be ashamed of, especially when it comes to a disease that is very well permanent. Family members, close friends, doctors, counselors, and even clergy members are good people to go to when talking is imperative.

Exercising when angry is not just for people in the movies. It actually helps to raise endorphins in the bloodstream and help people feel less stressed about their lives. Just being out in nature will help a person forget about the small things in life, and doing relaxing mind exercises while out in nature physically exercising is a good way to center the mind.

Lastly, taking time to relax and pamper one's self is not a shameful act. In fact, numerous people throughout the world would benefit from a spa day. Even just practicing muscle relaxation, meditation, visualization, and deep breathing in a comfortable setting will help. There are even public programs and classes that teach people how to relax.

There are so many consequences when it comes to being stressed long-term that it not only affects people with diabetes, but people without any other health concerns. Stress can lower the immune system, which is already compromised in people with diabetes, and it can increase heart rate. People with a constantly increased heart rate are at an even higher risk for heart disease, which is another complication of diabetes. Therefore, learning how to manage stress is imperative to being a healthy person.

Chapter 11 – Routine Management

A routine is nothing more than a set of habits performed on a repetitive basis. It takes thirty days plus to establish a routine, and even so, people may still forget things sometimes. To ensure a successful routine is established, it is best to use a calendar or even a phone app to remind the person when to take their medications, what they can and cannot eat, and when to test for blood sugar levels.

In order to create a routine, a diabetic must understand what affects their illness. Thing such as food, physical activity, medications, and emotional stability all can make diabetes either better or worse. Knowing what factors influence the blood glucose levels are imperative. Once a routine is established, it will lessen the risk for illness, stress, and hormone levels dropping or raising too high. Understanding the interactions of food and medication that the patient is taking are also very important. Remember, there are four different types of insulin and they are all taken at different times when it pertains to eating meals. Knowing which kind a person is taking is very important.

People with diabetes and people without this disease should have a schedule that revolves around their meals, physical activity, and sleep patterns. All human beings benefit from a comfortable routine that occurs daily. For people with diabetes, they must speak with their doctor about what time to take their insulin and start from there. Waking up at the same time daily will help the body regulate itself and it will be easier to keep a schedule for eating that first, important meal of the day, breakfast. Breakfast should be eaten at the same time, as well as the other important meals of the day, lunch and dinner.

Keeping a routine when it comes to physical activity will help regulate stress levels as well as hormone levels that may affect diabetics. Jogging or walking at the same time daily will create a sense of ease during the day. It is especially helpful to do this after something during the day that is stressful, such as arriving home from work after a long drive in traffic. Taking a walk will raise endorphins, which make people feel good. It also helps with memory, too, which helps in keeping a routine.

Activities that will maintain emotional stability are also very important. Meditating every morning or doing yoga in the evenings will help a person feel at peace. It is best to keep these activities healthy, so watching a favorite program on television is not considered appropriate. While it may reduce stress levels, it is not working out the body or the mind at the same time.

Conclusion

Hopefully, the information in this book will prove helpful when figuring out how to manage and cope with diabetes. Remember, always feel free to consult a professional about anything that may be worrisome, and keep a group of close friends and family members on call for when there might be an emotional need.

There is no need to stop living life to the fullest when living with diabetes. It's just a small bump in the road that will eventually become manageable. There are numerous people who live with the disease every day who are able to go on vacations, have fun, and hang out with friends and family just as they used to do before the diagnosis.